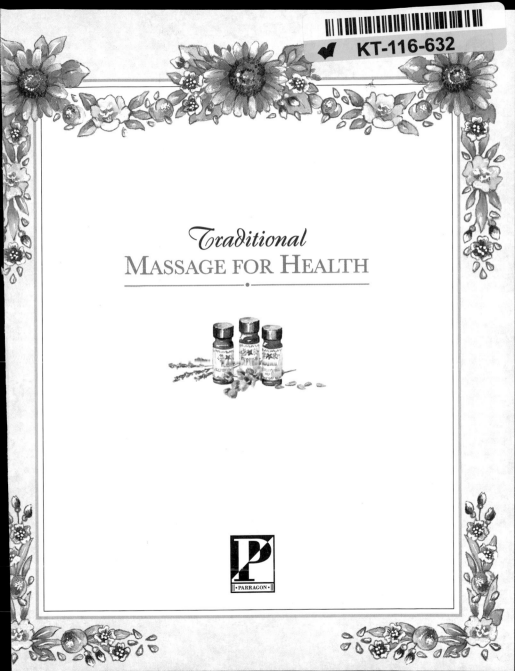

Traditional
MASSAGE FOR HEALTH

P

PARRAGON

Traditional
MASSAGE FOR HEALTH

EDITED BY MARGARET CROWTHER

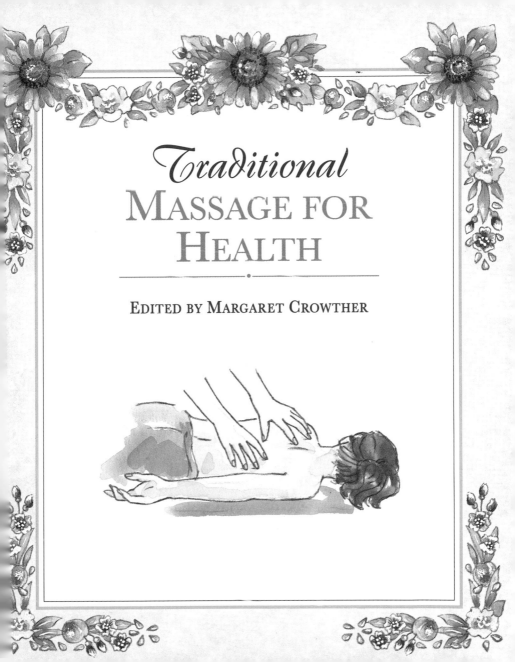

WARNING

If you have a medical condition, or are pregnant, the information in this book should not be followed without consulting your doctor first. All guidelines, warnings and instructions should be read carefully *before* embarking on any of the treatments. Although the treatments suggested in this book are unlikely to produce adverse side effects, there are always exceptions to the rule. The treatments are taken at the reader's sole discretion.

The publisher cannot accept responsibility for injuries or damage arising out of a failure to comply with the above.

First published in Great Britain in 1996 by
Parragon Book Service Ltd
Units 13-17, Avonbridge Industrial Estate
Atlantic Road, Avonmouth
Bristol BS11 9QD

© 1996 Parragon Book Service Ltd

ISBN 0-7525-1723-6

Printed in Great Britain
Produced by Kingfisher Design, London

Series Editor Jenny Plucknett
Series Design Pedro Prá-Lopez, Kingfisher Design

Massage consultant Alison J Wilkinson BABTAC IFA reg. Dip
Illustrations Jill Moore
Typesetting/DTP Frances Prá-Lopez, Kingfisher Design

Some of the material in this book has previously appeared in *Massage for Common Ailments* by Penny Rich, © 1994 Parragon Book Service Ltd

Contents

The Art of Massage 6

**Applying Massage
Techniques Safely** 8

CHAPTER 1
Basic Massage Techniques
First Requirements for Massage 10
Preparing for Massage 12
Massage Strokes
    Stroking 14
    Circling 15
    Friction Rub 16
    Kneading 17
    Raking......................................18
    Pummelling..............................19
    Knuckling 20
    Thumbing 21
    Stretching 22
    Pressing 23

CHAPTER 2
Therapeutic Massages
Massage for a Stiff Neck 24
Massage for a Tension Headache ..26
Massage for Lower Back Ache 28
Massage for Upper Back Ache 30

Massage for Aching
    Hands and Wrists 32
Massage for Aching Legs 35
Massage for Sore Feet 38

CHAPTER 3
Feel-good Massages
Fit for Life Massage.......................40
Energizing Body Massage..............42
The Circulation Booster 44

CHAPTER 4
Beautifying Massages
Beauty Massage for
    Face and Neck 46
Anti-stretch Mark Massage............49
Anti-cellulite Massage...................52

CHAPTER 5
**Massages for Special Health
    Problems**
Massage to Soothe Period Pains 54
Massage to Induce Sleep................56
Massage for Jetlag or Hangover 58
Massage to Soothe a Baby 60
Massage for a Child's
    Tummy Ache...........................62

Index 64

The Art of Massage

The art of massage is an ancient one. It has been practised for some 5000 years in the Middle and Far East, to cure and relieve many medical conditions, to relax the body and induce a feeling of calm and well-being, and to prevent disease by keeping the body in good condition.

MODERN MASSAGE TECHNIQUES

In the West, massage has evolved mainly from the work of the Swede, Per Henrik Ling, who developed and practised the techniques in the nineteenth century. Qualified masseurs have been trained in physiology and can give many specialized forms of treatment, but in its simplest form, massage is something anyone can learn to do, without special training. And giving someone a massage is a wonderful way to relax or re-energize them.

HOW MASSAGE CAN BE USED

Just as a parent rubs a child's hurting tummy, arm or leg to 'make it better', massage can soothe and help to cure a range of problems caused by damaged or over-used muscles and rheumatic conditions. But as well as soothing and relaxing painful muscles, ligaments and tendons it also stimulates the tissues and encourages good blood circulation, bringing oxygen-rich blood to the tissues and speeding up the removal of waste from the cells. This has a beneficial effect on both body and mind, soothing, relaxing, releasing tension, and generally promoting good health.

THE BENEFITS OF MASSAGE

The Ancient Greeks believed that a daily massage was one of the best ways of ensuring good health, and experts today agree that massage lowers blood pressure, improves body function and can help overcome pain and discomfort and generally speed up the healing process. Perhaps best of all, it is a simple, quick and sure way of bringing comfort and relaxation to a friend, child or partner and is pleasurable for the person doing the massage as well as for the person receiving it.

Applying Massage Techniques Safely

Repetitive strain injury, insomnia, fatigue, period pains, a child's tummy ache – these are just some of the conditions which can be relieved by massage, as described in the following chapters. Everyone from babies to grandparents can benefit, and the simple massage steps described in this book can be practised safely in almost all cases. But, as with anything, there are a few important do-s and don't-s.

WHAT NOT TO DO

❋ Never put heavy, downward pressure on bony areas (over spine, ribs, shoulders, shoulder blades, collar bone, elbows, knees).

❋ Never put heavy, downward pressure on organs (over the heart, abdomen, and small of the back where the kidneys are).

❋ If the person you are massaging so much as winces, stop immediately. Sometimes when you are massaging an area of knotted muscles it may be slightly painful, but the recipient should always feel it 'doing good'.

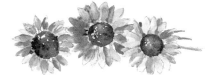

WHEN NOT TO MASSAGE

When massaging young children or elderly people, go extra gently; with a person who is ill or frail, do not massage without checking with a doctor first. Do not use massage during the first three months of pregnancy.

People with some conditions could be harmed by massage. Never massage anyone who has recently undergone surgery or anyone with any of the following conditions, unless advised by their doctor that it is safe:

* Skin infections or any contagious disease

* Cancer in any form

* Recent scar tissue

* High temperature or fever

* Epilepsy

* Varicose veins, phlebitis, thrombosis, or any heart or circulatory problems

* Asthma or any severe respiratory condition

* Recurrent or severe back pain

* Long-term injury

FOR YOUR OWN COMFORT

Massage can be almost as soothing and relaxing for the person giving it as for the person receiving it.

* Be aware of your posture so that you do not strain yourself.

* Lengthen your spine and neck with every movement.

* Do not hunch your shoulders.

* Keep your back flat as you bend forward.

* Stop immediately if any massage step is uncomfortable for you or causes you pain.

— 1 —

First Requirements for Massage

All you really need for massage is your hands and some massage oil. To ensure that your hands glide easily over the recipient's skin, oil them first, and re-oil them as you go, whenever you begin to feel the hands dragging rather than gliding. Mineral Oils are too thin, and some Vegetable Oils (Olive Oil, for example) are too heavy and sticky, but there is a wide range of inexpensive Vegetable, Nut and Flower Oils from which to choose. Some oils are more suitable for the body and others for the face but among these, you and the person being massaged may find you develop a personal preference. Choose from the oils listed opposite.

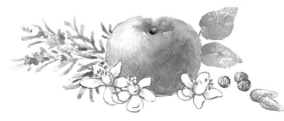

OILS FOR THE BODY

GRAPESEED • SAFFLOWER • SESAME SEED • SOYA • SUNFLOWER
SWEET ALMOND

OILS FOR THE FACE

APRICOT • AVOCADO • EVENING PRIMROSE • JOJOBA
PEACH KERNEL • SWEET ALMOND • WHEATGERM

PREPARING THE OIL

Make sure that your nails are short and then warm both your hands
and the oil before you start. Keep a small dish or a plastic,
flip-top container of the mixed oil nearby. To warm the oil,
put the container in a bowl of hot water for a few minutes.
You can use this hot water to dip your hands in too.

Preparing for Massage

The person being massaged needs to feel relaxed, so the first requirement is warmth and quiet. For many of the massage sequences in this book the person being massaged needs to be lying down. If you have a very firm bed, this can be used; but in most cases the floor will be better, and you will find that you can do the steps while kneeling next to the person on the floor. It is also possible to use a table, suitably covered, so that you can remain standing.

PADDING FOR COMFORT

You will need

❋ Plenty of padding material – a thick quilt, a futon or a foam mattress 5-8cm (2-3in) thick for the recipient to lie on and cushions for your own knees – to keep you both comfortable.

❋ A clean sheet to cover the surface to protect it from oil.

❋ Warm towels. These not only keep the massage recipient warm but you can use them to cover one part of the body while turning your attention to another. Towels are more convenient than blankets as, if they become oily, they can be washed. They can also be rolled to support the neck, put behind the knees when the person is lying face up and folded into a pad to place beneath the upper chest when you are working on the back.

SITTING UP

For massage sequences done with the recipient sitting up, he or she can either sit sideways on a chair with the head propped on a large cushion on a desk or on the back of a second chair, or the person can sit wrong way round on a chair, resting the head on a large cushion over the chair back.

GIVING THE MASSAGE

You will find that giving a massage is quite a warming experience, and you will be most comfortable wearing loose, cool clothes and keeping your feet bare. Some people like to talk while they are being massaged, while others fall into a deep, contented silence. As the person giving the massage, follow the recipient's lead, and talk only if he or she wants to. In some steps you will need to hold the position for a measured time – always count in your head, not out loud, for these holds.

MASSAGE STROKES

You need to master only a few techniques to give a full massage. Basically there are strokes that relax and strokes that stimulate. Most massage sequences begin and end with soothing stroking movements. The various techniques are described on pages 14-23.

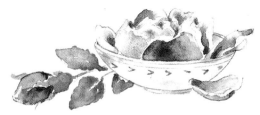

Stroking

The first and simplest movement, stroking, is done to warm and relax the tissue. Both hands are used palms down – held flat over large areas and curved for working on small areas. Stroking can also be done with fingers only, and you can 'cat stroke' with one hand following the other, using curved hands, so that only the fingertips are touching the skin at the end of the stroke. Always stroke smoothly and rhythmically, repeating the movements as much as you wish.

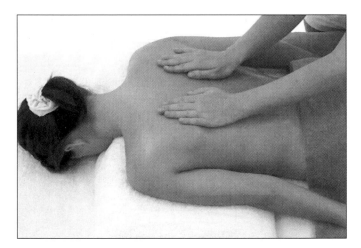

Circling

Circling is similar to stroking in its soothing effect. Both palms are used in just the same way, but as they stroke they move in circles, one clockwise and the other anti-clockwise. Sometimes, on large areas of muscle, circling is done more firmly with one hand placed over the other and the two hands together making a single circling movement. You can also use both hands to make one big sweeping circle, with each hand completing one half of the circle.

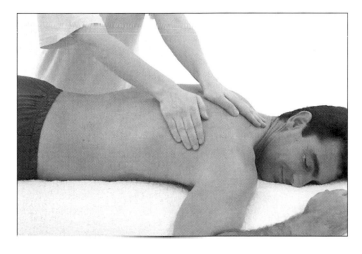

Friction Rub

This is a firmer stroke which stimulates the circulation and frees the joints. It is done with the hands held fairly stiffly, using the flat palms or just the stiffly held fingers and it can be done with the hands held sideways so that the sides of the little fingers do the work. The hands are moved back and forth along the skin in a sawing motion which is very warming.

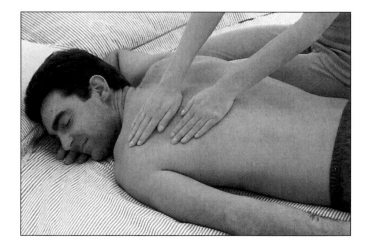

Kneading

This gives a firmer, stimulating massage to the larger muscles and begins with the hands placed palms down, fingers together and thumbs stretched out to the side. Use your thumbs to push into, squeeze and softly pinch the flesh up towards the fingers, moving your hands one after the other over the same area of the body. This is used to relax tense, contracted muscles and to treat deep tissue after the area has been relaxed and warmed by the earlier steps.

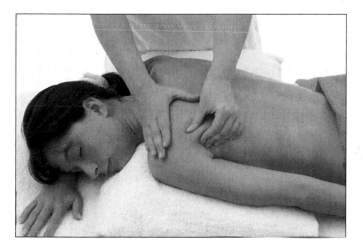

Raking

In raking, just the fingertips are used to rake over the skin in firm, pulling movements. You need to keep them stiffly bent at the joints and held so that only the fingertips touch the skin. Rake back towards you, using both hands together or pulling one hand after the other.

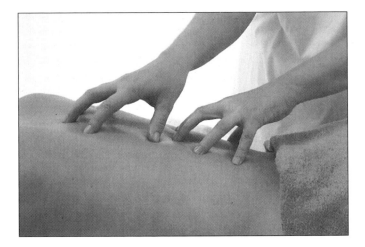

Pummelling

Pummelling is especially good at toning and stimulating fatty areas and is done with hands made into loose, relaxed fists. Bounce the fists rapidly up and down over areas being pummelled in a fast light drumming movement. You can pummel with hands held knuckles down, sideways, or palms upwards.

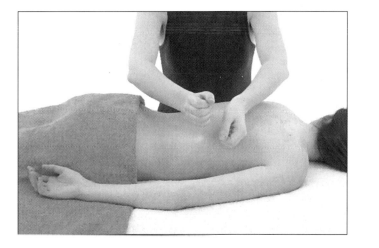

Knuckling

This is a firm but easy stroke made with the fingertips flat on the skin and moving in a rolling motion. Make your hands into lose fists and place them with the outer side of the fingertips flat on the skin. Roll them forward, turning them right over so that the knuckles push and slide into the skin. You can also do the stroke with the palms upwards, lightly rubbing your knuckles across the skin.

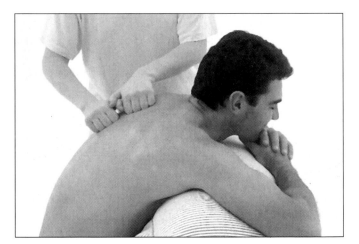

Thumbing

For this stroke, use the pads and sides of your thumbs to knead or deeply stroke into the flesh. You can also use the thumb tips to make circling motions, or to push down, hold, then release over deep muscle tissue. This is an excellent way of stimulating and relaxing the muscles up either side of the spine.

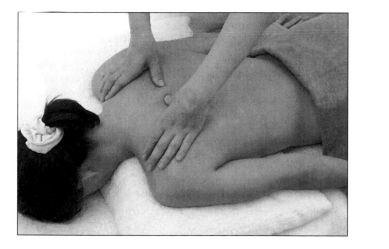

Stretching

This stroke exerts a firm downward pressure of the hands as you slide them apart in opposite directions to pull and stretch the skin and underlying muscles. Use palms held flat for this stroke. On arms and legs you can also twist and wring (gently) as you stretch, by turning the hands in opposite directions.

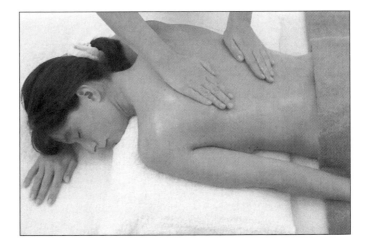

Pressing

Pressing is a good way to finish off any of the other strokes, to reinforce the effect and help to release muscle tension. Press using the heels of your hands, or, for small areas, use just your index fingers. For large muscles, place one palm on top of the other for a stronger press and press down firmly for a count of 10.

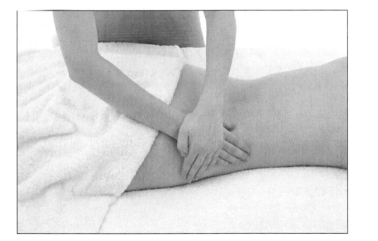

— 2 —

Massage for a Stiff Neck

Tension, bad posture, draughts, sleeping on the wrong kind of pillow – all can cause a stiff neck. Luckily, massage can bring relief, and it can even be done, say in an office, with the sufferer sitting fully clothed in a chair and leaning forward over a desk, resting her head on a cushion. Simple movements, with lots of warming repetitions, are what's needed, with some deep kneading strokes to relax and release trapped nerves and muscle tension.

Quantity of oil required: 5ml (1 tsp) of an oil for the face or body, *see page 11*

1 With flats of hands on either side of the spine, repeatedly stroke firmly from middle to top of back.(Do not massage the spine itself.) At the shoulders, slide out to the tops of the arms then back along tops of shoulders and up sides of neck. Then, using the sides of the hands and holding hands straight, do a firm, fast friction massage along right shoulder muscle from arm to neck. Repeat on the left side.

2 Using your thumbs only, knead under the shoulder blades and up the sides of the spine to the top of the neck in small circular movements. Spread your hands, one each side, over the shoulder muscles by the sides of the neck and push and pull the muscles back and forth.

3 Work on each side separately, with both hands, squeezing, pinching, and kneading the shoulder muscles. Finish by sweeping the palms one after the other from the top of the arm and up the side of the neck, working from the opposite side.

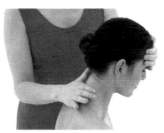

4 With the person sitting up, support her forehead with your palm and with the other hand massage quickly up and down the neck in a light friction stroke. Follow by rolling the hand lightly from side to side across the neck to push and pull the muscles against the vertebrae. Finally place your thumb and finger either side of the top vertebra. Press.

Hold for a count of 10. Release, and make small circles over the area. Circle in this way across the base of the skull from ear to ear.

5 Cup her arm tops with your hands and gently push the shoulders forward until you feel a stretch. Hold for 10. Stretch the shoulders back and hold in the same way without moving your hands. Then place the palms of your hands on the tops of the shoulders, either side of the neck. Press firmly down while the sufferer leans her head back as far as comfortable. Hold for 10. Relax as she raises her head.

6 Support the right side of her head just above the ear as you bend her head to the right. Place your left hand below her left ear with fingers stretched and slide your hand repeatedly down the length of the neck and across the shoulder top to the arm, pressing down to stretch the muscle. Repeat on the other side.

Massage for a Tension Headache

A slow and gentle scalp massage can help to soothe away a headache and leaves you feeling calm and tranquil after a busy day. For a headache or migraine, give lots of slow, soothing strokes, and concentrate on areas where you can feel tension. A neck massage, see pages 24-25, will help too. The aim is to relax, so the person being massaged should be lying comfortably on her back.

Quantity of oil required: 5ml (1tsp) of an oil for the face, *see page 11*

WARNING

If you have frequent or severe headaches, consult your doctor

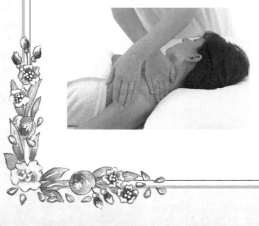

1 Using the palms (*left*), pull one hand after the other rhythmically along one shoulder muscle from arm to ear in a firm, stroking movement. Repeat on the other shoulder.

2 Slide your hands under the back and pull up from low between the shoulder blades to the nape of the neck. Let one hand follow the other and use a

firm stroke. Then place the hands under the nape of the neck and, with flat fingertips, gently stretch the neck. When you feel resistance hold for 5. (Do not raise the head.) Do this smoothly, three times.

3 Cup the face in your hands and gently pull up the sides of the cheeks, pressing in over the temples. When your hands meet above the eyebrows draw palms in turn up to the hairline. Press top and sides of head and hold for 5.

4 With fingertips, make tiny circles all round the hairline to rotate the scalp for a count of 10. Keep the fingers stiff and use light pressure. Work back to crown and around nape of neck. Then very gently tug sections of hair to relax the scalp, holding it close to the roots. Finally push in with your hands and squeeze the head all over.

5 With fingers, gently press on the eyelids for a count of 5 and repeat twice. With tips of first two fingers, stroke the eyebrows firmly,

working outwards, then make slow circles over the temples working from brows up to the hairline.

6 Return to the shoulders and cup shoulders at tops of arms. Gently press down and hold for 5, twice. Slide hands under, push the shoulders upwards, rounding them into the chest to release upper back and neck support muscles. Hold for 5 and repeat.

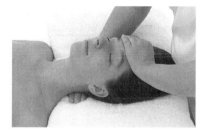

7 With right palm under back of neck and left palm on forehead, slowly draw both hands towards crown, pushing gently inwards. The lower hand should gently lift and tilt the head. Repeat several times.

Massage for Lower Back Ache

Two out of three people suffer from back ache at some time in their lives. While it can be brought on by lifting a heavy object, or by pregnancy, it can also begin with something as silly as a sudden sneeze. Plenty of muscle-toning exercise can help to prevent back problems, as can sensible lifting and carrying. (Bend the legs when lifting so as not to strain the back.) Luckily, massage is a great cure for back ache.

The person being massaged should be lying comfortably, face-down on a well-padded floor or firm mattress, with a rolled towel placed under the upper chest and neck so that the head is in a relaxed, face-down position. Strokes should be slow and rhythmic, with lots of repetitions. The person giving the massage should stand or kneel level with the tops of the thighs of the person being massaged.

Quantity of oil required: 5ml (1tsp) of an oil for the body, *see page 11*

1 Starting at the base of the spine, with the palms about 5cm (2in) either side of the spine, slide hands lightly up to the waist, then fan them out to the sides in one smooth movement. Massage more firmly down, across the buttocks, to the spine base. Repeat several times.

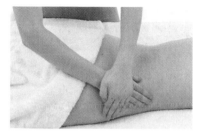

3 Reach to the far side of lower back and tuck the fingers of one hand under the top of the thigh. With fingers firm, pull flesh up towards spine. Follow with second hand in same position and repeat so that hands follow each other in a firm, stroking motion. Work up from hip to waist and repeat on the other side of the torso.

2 Palms down, overlap hands, and gently make slow circles all over buttocks and lower back muscles from waist to tail bone to warm and relax. Keep fingers flat but relaxed so that pressure comes from the heel of the palms. (Do not massage the spine itself.) Follow with light thumbing strokes in small circles radiating out from each side of the spine and up, moving from tailbone to waist. Start 5cm (2in) from each side of spine and repeat, working further out towards the hips each time. Pressure can be firmer over knotted areas as long as it does not hurt.

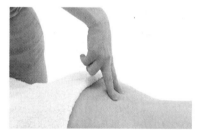

4 Finally run the stiffly held first two fingers of one hand right down the spine, 5cm (2in) apart on each side, from nape of neck to tailbone, and then repeat Step 1.

Massage for Upper Back Ache

Upper back ache is likely to be caused by tension and bad posture – standing all day, or sitting over a word processor, and even slouching in an easy chair. The upper back massage can be combined with the lower back massage, see pages 28-29, for an all-in-one therapeutic and relaxing routine that will help to prevent back trouble as well as to cure it. Have the person being massaged lying face down, and use slow, light, rhythmic strokes with lots of smooth repetitions.

Quantity of oil required: 5ml (1tsp) of an oil for the body, *see page 11*

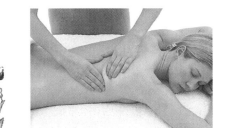

1 Place palms below the waist on either side of the spine, 5cm (2in) away, and slide them lightly up and out to the shoulders and back more firmly down the sides to the starting position. Then, with a gentle pinching movement of the thumbs and fingers, (*left*) lightly knead over the soft tissue of the back

from waist to shoulders, working with both hands together. Concentrate on relaxing tight, knotty areas at the shoulder tops and avoid the spine and any bony parts.

tops at the sides of the neck, fingers resting on collar bone. Pull firmly back, with an inward pressure, one hand after the other. Then with both hands squeeze and knead each shoulder muscle, in turn, from top of arm to neck.

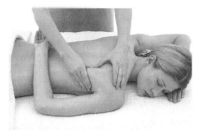

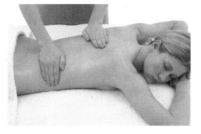

2 To make the shoulder bone jut out, bend the person's arm and place the hand, palm up, on the lower back. Knead around the shoulder blade, with deep, flicking thumb movements. Follow with small thumbed circles and finish with long, slow strokes with the sides of the thumbs.

3 Pull and stretch the muscles along the tops of the shoulders, starting with hands cupped over the shoulder

4 Hold the tops of the arms and gently pull back the shoulders until they are slightly raised. Hold for 10, lower and repeat. Then place palms down over the spine in the middle of the back and glide hands apart diagonally, pulling crosswise to stretch the skin and muscles from hip to opposite shoulder (*above*). Hold for 10. Repeat on the opposite side.

Massage for Aching Hands and Wrists

Tension and demanding manual work, including repetitive light movements – working on a keyboard or knitting, for example – can lead to aching hands and wrists. Gentle flexes and finger strokes release tension and soothe tender areas, and this massage also brings relief to arthritic and rheumatic aches and pains.

Use plenty of oil, keep the thumb strokes light and gentle to soothe rather than stimulate, and never take the stretches beyond the point of comfort. Soaking the person's hands in warm water for 10 minutes first helps to make the massage more beneficial. Work on each hand in turn, repeating all the steps. You can adapt this massage to work on your own hands.

Quantity of oil required: 5ml (1tsp) of an oil for the body, *see page 11*

1 Using both hands, grasp the thumb and little finger of the person's hand firmly between your ring and little fingers. Push down to open up the person's palm.

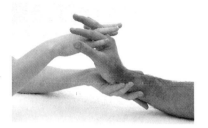

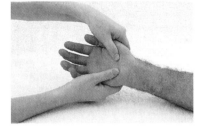

hands – your fingers curved over to his palms. Slide the heels of your hands apart to roll his hand under and stretch it across the back. Hold for 10. Release and repeat.

2 Support the forearm in the palm of one hand and interlock the fingers of your other hand through the fingers of the person being massaged. Holding your fingers stiffly, gently push up your hand to stretch the person's hand from wrist to fingertips. Push back from tips, not base, of the person's fingers, and do not over-extend the stretch. Hold for 15. Release. Then, still supporting the forearm, lay your palm over his knuckles, fingers pointing up the arm, and flex the hand by gently pushing down with the heel of your hand into the first joints of his fingers. Hold for 15. Release.

3 With your wrists together, wrap the back of his hand with your

4 Turn his hand over, tuck your fingers under the back of his hand and pick it up. Make small circles over the palm, using your thumbs only, in a light, gliding stroke. Next use the sides of your thumbs to do long straight strokes along the palm from wrists to fingers. Then slide your hands along until your thumbs are over the inner wrist and do very light strokes along both sides of the tendon, for about 5cm (2in), then fan out to each side.

continued overleaf

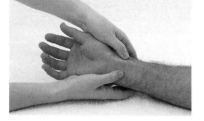 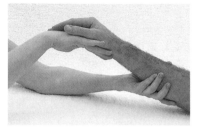

5 Encircle the wrist with the thumb and first two fingers of both hands, and move one hand clockwise while the other goes anti-clockwise in a light wringing motion.

6 Support the person's forearm in the palm of your hand again and slide the other hand up under his palm. Push your fingers forward to interlock with his, and by pulling them back up toward you, lightly stroke repeatedly between his fingers up to the nails. Finish by sandwiching the hand between your hands, and pressing lightly to a count of 10.

Massage for Aching Legs

With every step each leg in turn takes the weight of your entire body, and even if you sit all day, your legs can get tense and tired. Aching legs affect your whole body and can also lead to such problems as varicose veins and oedema (swelling). Leg massage helps relax the muscles and boost the blood circulation, giving you renewed energy.

Firm upward strokes and fast friction rubs are best. The person being massaged should lie, face down, on a firm surface either on the floor or high enough for you to stand comfortably. Use plenty of massage oil, and keep each leg covered, in turn, while you work on the other. After the massage the person should rest for 10 minutes with the feet propped up on pillows or against a wall, so that they are higher than the head.

Quantity of oil required: 5-10ml (1-2tsp) of an oil for the body, *see page 11*

1 Place the palms each side of one ankle, fingers pointing up the leg, just above the bone. Push up the sides of the leg, pressing in firmly with the heel of the hand and keeping the fingers relaxed. Release pressure at knee area and press in again towards tops of thighs. Massage lightly back down the leg, stretching the skin back towards the foot. Then stretch the back of the leg by gently bending the heel up towards the bottom as far as is comfortable. Hold for 5. Repeat.

continued overleaf

2 Press with your thumbs on the outer sides of the leg above the ankle bone and slowly slide them upward, along the calf muscle, to the knee. Thumb-stroke the whole calf from outer to inner leg, working in upward lines.

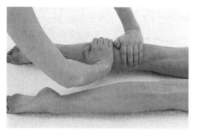

3 Place hands, palms down and one below the other with fingers pointing in opposite directions, across the calf muscle just below the knee. With firm pressure, slide them up to the top of the thigh in one long stroke, fan out and draw them back with lighter pressure. Bend back the heel and hold, as in Step 1.

4 Knead the back of the thigh muscle all over, pinching between thumb and fingers of both hands and pressing deeply into the muscle. Knead sides of the thigh with fingers curved around the leg. Finish with two more knee to thigh palm strokes as in Step 3.

5 Place the hands with wrists together, and fingers wrapped round the leg at lower calf. Press down the heels of the hands and slide the hands out and away around the leg, pushing the flesh towards the front of the leg. Continue up the calf to just below the knee and then from above knee to top of thigh.

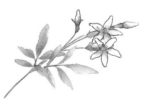

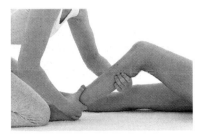

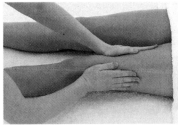

6 Turn over the person being massaged and bend her knee, holding her foot between your knees. Above the ankle, curve your hands around the back of the leg, one hand above the other, thumbs towards the front. With firm pressure push one hand after the other from ankle to knee. Fan out at the top and firmly palm stroke back down sides of the calf. Finish stroke by gripping the ankle firmly. Repeat up the back and down the front of the thigh, from just above the knee, with each hand in turn.

7 Straighten the leg. Work palms in a backwards and forwards sawing motion up the sides of the leg from ankle to thigh. Bend the leg and repeat with one hand at the front and the other at the back of the leg. Repeat the sequence from Step 1 on the other leg. Finish by holding the ankles and pulling gently to extend the legs for a count of 10. Release and repeat.

Massage for Sore Feet

Most of us ignore our feet or take them for granted until they let us down. Yet when they do, they certainly let us know about it. A soothing massage can soon sort out troublesome feet, but there is no need to wait until something goes wrong. A good massage not only gets rid of aches – it also helps to keep the feet flexible and healthy to lighten your step and improve your mood.

Feet are very sensitive. They have 38 muscles and 28 bones, as well as innumerable nerve endings branching out from the body's main nerves. So it is hardly surprising that a foot massage can be a tonic for the whole body. Use plenty of oil for this massage, and work gently on the bony top of the foot, more firmly on the sole. Follow the steps through first on one foot and then on the other.

Quantity of oil required: 5ml (1 tsp) of an oil for the body, *see page 11*

1 Start with a friction rub, rubbing the whole foot briskly between your palms. Prop the foot across your leg and rub up and down the heel with hands parallel to the calf. Then place one hand on the back of the heel and the other over the front of

the ankle so that the foot is sandwiched between your palms and give long slow strokes from ankle to toes. Follow the contours of the foot in firm flowing strokes.

2 Lift the foot, with the left hand behind the ankle, and place the palm of your right hand flat against the sole. Push in to follow the contours closely and gently push against the toes to flex back the foot. Hold for 10. Repeat four times.

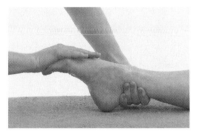

3 Place the palm of your left hand round the back of the ankle, to support the foot, and wrap your right palm over the toes with the thumb under the sole of the foot. Gently push the toes downwards. Hold for 10. Repeat four times, then gently push the foot from side to side five times.

4 Wrap the fingers of both hands round the top of the foot and make small circles with your thumbs across the sole from toes to heel. When you reach the heel, push and stroke back to the toes, keeping the thumbs stiff. Repeat thumb circling and stroking in the same way on the upper part of the foot with your fingers wrapped under the foot at the arches and using only light pressure.

5 Rest the foot on your leg and hold it firmly over the arch with your left hand to massage the toes. Rub, pull and gently rotate each toe in turn, working up to the tip.

6 Finally, hold the back of the ankle firmly with your right hand, squeezing the tendon behind the ankle bone. With the left hand, palm down across the instep, stroke towards the toes in a firm flowing movement getting slower and lighter to finish the massage.

— 3 —
Fit for Life Massage

Experts now say that about 15 minutes daily exercise will delay body ageing by ten to twenty years. The fit-for-life massage helps to keep you moving by boosting circulation and working on the muscles that seize up most quickly. It is never too late, or too soon, to begin – this massage suits children and the over-70s alike.

Quantity of oil required: 10ml (2tsp) of an oil for the body, *see page 11*

1 With the person being massaged lying face down, first give a fast, all-over friction rub. Work up over feet, legs, buttocks and back, then hands and arms. Use palms, sides of hands, heels of hands and stiff fingertips, interchangeably. Then, with a pummelling stroke, bounce hands off skin working upward as before, from soles of feet to upper back and shoulders. Use flat fists, knuckles, base of fists or flicking fingers. Be firm with large muscles and light on bony or sensitive areas.

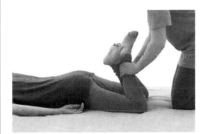

the knees towards the chest. Hold, release and repeat as in Step 2.

5 With the legs stretched straight out, firmly grasp both feet and toes from above and gently stretch the legs. Count to 15, release and repeat. Move round and stretch the arms in the same way, keeping them raised at a 45° angle.

2 Cross the person's ankles, slowly take feet towards buttocks and stop when you feel resistance. Hold for 15, release. Drop the feet back to the floor and repeat twice. (This must not cause discomfort.)

3 Lightly place your hands, palm down, in the middle of the back. Slide one hand towards one side of the hips and the other towards the opposite shoulder. Stretch between your hands for a count of 10. Repeat in reverse; then stretch one hand up to the neck and the other down to the tailbone twice in the same way.

4 With the person on her back, cross her ankles and gently bend

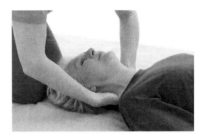

6 To round off, interlock your fingers under the nape of the person's neck and gently lift, stretch and arch the neck, keeping the top of the head on the floor. Hold for 10. If you wish, finish with an all-over massage as in the first part of Step 1.

Energizing Body Massage

Many of us lead busy lives which tire us more mentally than physically. The result is often that we sleep badly and then feel more tired still, yet we have to force ourselves to keep going and the effects of stress build up. This massage is one of the best gifts you could make to a friend or partner – it rubs away the physical signs of stress and releases muscle tension, invigorating both body and mind.

The person being massaged should sit bent forwards onto a pillow resting on a desk or propped against a chair-back. Bare skin is best, but the massage can also be done while the person is still clothed.

Quantity of oil required: 5ml (1tsp) of an oil for the body, *see page 11*

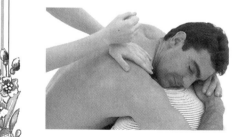

1 Holding one hand, palm down, on the upper back, make a firm fist with the other hand and bounce it up and down over the flat hand. Move all over the upper back in this way for several minutes vibrating the muscles. Avoid the spine. Then lightly slap over the area with your little fingers and tips of middle and ring fingers in a quick up and down stroke.

2 Knead the shoulder muscles by squeezing between your fingers and thumbs. Then place your forearms on the shoulders, with your hands hanging relaxed to the front, and gently lean down, using your body-weight to press down the shoulder tops in a comfortable stretch. Hold for 10. Relax. Push the shoulders forward, holding the arm tops. Hold, release, and pull back, to stretch.

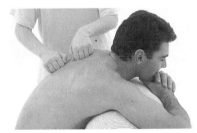

3 5cm (2in) away from one side of the spine roll your knuckles across and down the long back muscle from nape of neck to buttock. Use firm fists and press into the muscle as you roll your hands forward. At the bottom, repeat on the other side.

4 Place palms firmly on the lower back, 5cm (2in) either side of the spine, and slide one hand up and the other hand down in slow, firm strokes. Gradually work up to shoulder tops, stretching and pulling the skin in opposite directions. Then, with the person more upright, support his head with your left palm as you knead from the nape of the neck up to the base of the skull with thumb and fingers placed either side of the vertebrae. Finish by making small circles over this area with your thumbs.

5 With stiff, straight fingers, rake and gently scrub all over the scalp from the hairline to the crown. Then make long firm strokes all over the head. Finally use flat, loose fingers to slap and tap the head lightly in a fast up-and-down movement.

6 End the massage with a light finger chop across the shoulder tops, bouncing the sides of the hands rapidly up and down first on one shoulder then on the other.

The Circulation Booster

This massage boosts the circulation to the extremities. But while it is a boon for people who have cold hands and feet, everyone benefits from the way it stimulates blood flow so that fresh, oxygen-rich blood circulates the body and wastes are rapidly flushed away.

The best way to do the massage is for the recipient to lie on the floor or on a firm, low bed, while you kneel beside her. Keep the rest of the body covered while you are working on each area, so that all the body warmth is kept in.

Quantity of oil required: 10ml (2tsp) of an oil for the body, *see page 11*

1 Sandwich the right foot between your palms and give the foot a fast, firm friction rub. Continue for several minutes, then stroke the foot gently but firmly from toes to ankle, keeping it between your palms.

2 Raise the leg and support it at the ankle with your right hand. Push your left hand firmly up from ankle to knee. After six strokes repeat with the

other hand. Repeat this step twice more, then lower the leg.

3 Give a fast friction rub of the thigh with both palms, followed by slow, firm strokes with the heel of the hand, keeping the fingers relaxed and curved. Repeat these steps on the other foot and leg.

4 Raise the person's left arm from the elbow and hold her forearm at

the wrist with your thumb over her pulse. With light finger and thumb pressure, slide the other hand down the lower arm. Swap hands and massage the arm in this way, continuously swapping hands in a flowing movement for several minutes. Repeat on the other arm.

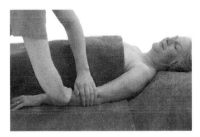

5 With her arm by her side place your palms over her wrist, pointing in opposite directions. Push both hands up the arm to the shoulder, slowly and deeply. Curve your top hand over the top of the shoulder and then slide both hands lightly back down the length of the arm to the fingers. Repeat rhythmically for several minutes and then repeat on the other arm.

6 With the person being massaged turned to face down, place your palms on the soles of her feet, fingers facing inwards. Slowly and firmly push the hands up over the heels, up the calf, gently over the backs of the knees, and more firmly up the thighs and sides of buttocks to the hips. Repeat ten times.

7 Kneel by her waist and do a full arm stroke on the backs of the arms starting with your palms over the backs of her hands, fingers pointing upwards. Push slowly up the arms with medium pressure, gently over the backs of the elbows and more firmly to the tops of the arms and across the shoulders to the neck. Repeat ten times with even pressure.

8 Sandwich each hand in turn between your palms and give a firm, fast friction rub from fingers to wrist for several minutes. Finally squeeze each hand between your palms for a count of 10, then slowly slide your fingers down and away from her finger tips.

— 4 —

Beauty Massage for Face and Neck

Massaging the face releases all the tiny muscles that give facial expression and can have an instantaneous beautifying effect, making your face look smoother and more relaxed. It does not actually exercise the muscles, and so it cannot prevent wrinkles or act as a natural facelift, but it does beat tension and make you look serene, and of course you can massage yourself.

Quantity of oil required: 5ml (1tsp) of an oil for the face, *see page 11*

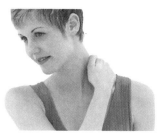

1 With palms, stroke face out from chin, over jawbone and cheeks and in to eyebrows. Press closed eyes with fingertips and count to 10. Repeat. With alternating palms, firmly stroke from eyebrows to hairline. Repeat. Then massage neck firmly from shoulder to ear (*left*), using right hand for left side and vice versa.

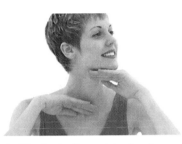

2 Rhythmically work backs of hands alternately up from collarbone and across jaw towards opposite ears, then lightly pat chin and jawline from side to side with backs of fingers in quick flicking movements. Drop back head, stretch neck and count to 5.

3 Run index fingers down sides of nose and around nostrils. Firmly press into middle of top lip. Repeat. Run first two fingers of one hand down the bridge of the nose, opening round nostrils and meeting in middle of top lip. Repeat.

4 Stroke firmly up the forehead from bridge of nose with first two fingers of each hand in turn. Then, working outwards, stroke along brows several times with middle two fingers (*above*). Gently press inner eye corners with thumbs, count to 4, and work round eye sockets in small pressing steps, changing to index fingers to work back under eyes. Press at inner corners.

continued overleaf

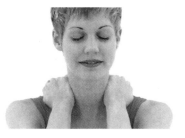

6 Stroke the face from chin to temples (*below left*) as in Step 1, but finish the stroke at the brows, then palm firmly up the forehead with each hand in turn. Press the temples with the first two fingers of each hand, and with the same pressure move the fingers on the spot in small circles. Hold, press and count to 10.

5 Drop head and chin and massage across shoulder muscles with fingertips, in circular movements from neck outwards. Then drop back head and pinch, knead and squeeze shoulder muscles. Press firmly with palms at sides of neck and repeat A E I O U out loud, to relax the jaw and neck.

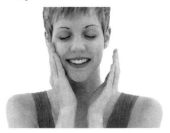

7 Use one hand, fingers held stiff, to make figure of 8 movements, stroking from between brows, out, round, up, above each eye in turn. Then lightly pat both sides of the face with flats of the hands (*above*). Press palms against sides of face for a count of 10. Relax and hold.

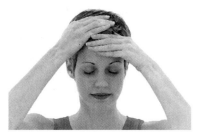

Anti-stretch Mark Massage

Stretch marks are usually caused by the skin stretching during pregnancy. To help prevent them, Steps 1-4 should be done during pregnancy and Steps 5-8 as a post-natal massage. Use plenty of Wheatgerm, Jojoba or Sweet Almond oil. The person being massaged should lie face up, but later in pregnancy she may find it more comfortable to turn on her side and lie with her knees bent.

Do not massage during the first three months of preganancy. When giving the massage, use lots of oil and keep all the movements on the tummy as light and gentle as possible.

Quantity of oil required: 10ml (2tsp) of an oil for the body, *see page 11*

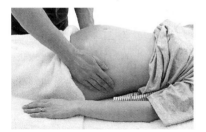

1 Start with hands over the solar plexus pointing up the chest and draw your palms gently out to the sides, pull fairly firmly down the sides of the waist and gently over the hips to below the navel. Repeat continuously to warm and spread the oil.

continued overleaf

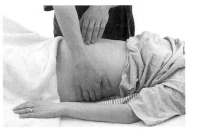

4 Lightly make large clockwise circles round the abdomen from the solar plexus – first using one hand, then with one hand following the other in a flowing motion.

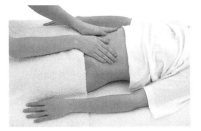

2 Firmly stroke up the sides of the waist. With both hands palm down against one thigh, and fingers tucked down under the bottom, pull the hands up the sides of the torso one after the other in smooth, flowing strokes. Repeat on the other side.

3 Bend one leg up at the knee and with both hands do firm, sweeping strokes up to the knee. Then, from above the knee, move along the thigh on inner and outer sides, taking the outer strokes up to the hip. Repeat on the other leg.

5 Place hands below navel with thumbs together and palms slightly raised so that only the fingers touch the tummy. Gently slide upwards and glide out towards the sides, pulling firmly down the sides of the waist and gliding lightly back to the starting position. Repeat this step several times.

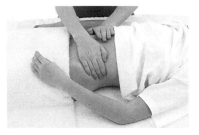

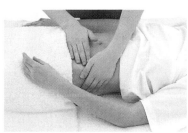

6 Place hands, palms down, one each side of the waist. Pull them again and again firmly up the sides and across the tummy to the opposite sides, criss-crossing them over the abdomen.

8 Place your hands centrally on the abdomen, one just below the ribs and the other below the navel. Circle round in a clockwise direction, with the first hand beginning the circle and the second hand completing it in one flowing stroke.

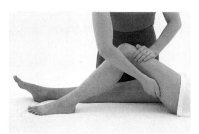

7 With the leg bent at the knee slide your right hand firmly up the thigh muscle to the buttock. Repeat on the other leg.

Anti-cellulite Massage

Cellulite is a word used by the beauty industry to describe the dimpled, orange-peel flesh that all too easily accumulates on thighs and buttocks. The current theory is that it is a sign that toxic wastes are lurking in fatty cells in those areas as a result of poor circulation, linked to lack of exercise. Massage can help to improve circulation, to flush away wastes and leave the skin tingling and rosy.

For best results have a do-it-yourself massage morning and night, using plenty of oil or body lotion, and do all the strokes upwards, towards the heart. Naturally it makes good sense to have plenty of exercise too, and limit your intake of tea, coffee, alcohol and sugary and fatty food.

Quantity of oil required: 10ml (2tsp) of an oil for the body, *see page 11*

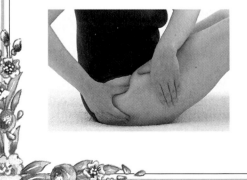

1 Sitting on the floor with legs bent at the knee, stroke firmly up the thigh from knee to top, one hand after the other in a flowing motion. Cover front, inner side, back and outer side. Then knead the thigh firmly all over, using both hands and squeezing the flesh between thumb and fingers, again working from knee up (*left*).

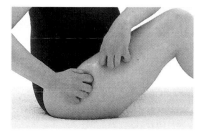

down and round from the hip. Then knead the buttock muscle, pinching flab firmly and briskly with thumb and fingers, from the curve of the buttock up towards the hip.

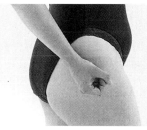

2 Bend your fingers stiffly and firmly drag both hands from knee up, rolling the hands under so that the knuckles also rake the skin, one hand following the other. Next with loose, relaxed fists pummel lightly all over the thigh tapping down and bouncing quickly back up.

4 Pummel the buttock with the hand in a loose, relaxed fist, working in an upwards direction. Finish off with long, smooth, deep strokes with the palms, using one hand after the other, from mid-thigh, up over the buttock to the hip. Repeat all the steps on the other thigh and buttock.

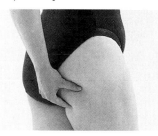

3 Stand up to treat the buttocks. Make large firm, flowing circles over your right buttock with the flat of your right hand, working clockwise

— 5 —
Massage to Soothe Period Pains

While massage may not completely dispel period pains
it can reduce the bloated feeling in your abdomen and soothe
the cramps and lower back ache. All the strokes should be light,
gentle and soothing, with plenty of repeats. If you have back
pain and feel you need a firmer massage get your friend
or partner to follow the instructions for lower
back ache given on pages 28-29.

Quantity of oil required: 5ml (1tsp) of an oil for the body, *see page 11*

1 The person being massaged
should be lying face down.
Place your hands 5cm (2in)
either side of the tail bone. Push
them up, fan smoothly out to the
sides at the waist, pull them
down the torso and back across
the buttocks, pulling and pushing
the flesh up, round and down.

2 Starting with the hands each
side of the top of the waist,
use the heels of the palms and
little fingers to press firmly,
sliding the hands down to the
hips, drawing in to the sides of
the spine. Slide them up the
middle of the back and fan them
out over the top of the waist.

3 Use the heel of the right
hand to stroke in circles over
the tailbone. Then place the
heels of both hands one each side

of the tailbone, and slowly push up each side of the spine to the waist and glide lightly back down.

4 Make small circles up the lower back from tailbone to waist (still 5cm (2in) away from spine). Then place your hands under the hips and pull up the flesh with your fingers forwards, towards the middle of the lower back in smooth, repetitive strokes.

5 Using thumbs and fingers of both hands knead each side of the torso from thigh top to waist, gently pinching, twisting and squeezing. Then repeat the same kneading process across the tops of the buttocks and up the middle of the lower back to the waist.

6 With the person turned face up, hold one hand in place over the solar plexus. Place the other palm above the navel and lightly make large clockwise circles down one side, across the groin and up to the starting position. Keep the stroke very light.

7 Place both hands over the solar plexus with the fingers pointing upwards. Slowly fan the hands out to the sides, and firmly down the waist. Sweep them round under the navel and gently slide them up to the starting position.

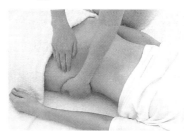

8 Place both hands on one side of the waist, with the fingers tucked well under the back. Firmly pull up the flesh towards the navel, one hand after the other, from the top of the thigh to the top of the waist. Gently bend up the person's knees to her chest with your hands pressing on the tops of her shins and hold for 10.

Massage to Induce Sleep

Insomnia is irritating and frustrating – for the parent or partner, as well as for the person who is unable to sleep. A warm bath followed by a long, slow massage loosens and relaxes knotted muscles and banishes tension, so that everyone can get to sleep! This massage is best done in bed, with light rhythmic strokes and plenty of repetitions. The person being massaged should lie face down.

Quantity of oil required: 10ml (2tsp) of an oil for the body, *see page 11*

1 Sit or kneel by the insomniac's legs and place your hands over the backs of his ankles, fingers pointing inwards. Quickly slide your hands to the tops of the thighs in one smooth stroke. Repeat several times. Then cross his feet at the heels, and slowly bend them towards his bottom as far as feels easy. Hold for 15. Release and repeat. Slowly friction rub calves and thighs, moving your hands in a sawing motion across the legs.

2 Cover up the lower body and kneel by the hips. Starting with hands on the lower back, pointing towards the spine, make a firm stroke right up the back and fan out your hands at the shoulders, turning them to pull down the arms.

3 Return to any knotted areas and knead deeply, squeezing the flesh between the fingers and thumbs. Tops of shoulders and lower back are likely trouble spots. Then make small, circular thumb strokes under the shoulder blades and up the nape of the neck.

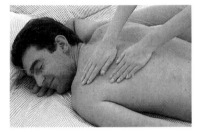

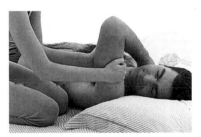

4 Keeping your hands parallel, give a sweeping friction rub with your palms. Go up and down from the lower back to the shoulder tops, each side of the spine, fast at first, then increasingly slowly. Each stroke should be about 20cm (8in) long.

5 With the person face up and the upper body covered, hold one foot around the top of the instep, prop it against your knee or thigh and gently push up the toes to flex it backward. Hold for 5. Release. Then move the toes from side to side and make slow circles with them in the air.

6 Place the palms at the tops of the thighs and stroke firmly down to the toes in one continuous movement. Then hold the feet firmly at the backs of the ankles and gently stretch the legs.

7 Interlock fingers, holding the person's hand palm to palm. Push his hand gently back and forward to flex and stretch it. Then hold his upper arm between your hands (*above*) and lift it, letting the elbow bend and the hand relax. Push in and squeeze with the heels and palms of your hands all the way down the arm to the wrist, avoiding the elbow. End by placing both hands around the arm top and slide them down to the wrist. Hold the hand and gently pull to lengthen the arm. Repeat on other arm.

8 Turn the person's head to one side and stroke the shoulder, up the side of the neck, over the jaw and cheek to the temple, with one hand following the other. Lift the head and

Massgage for Jetlag or a Hangover

This is a soothing massage that will make the person suffering from the night before better able to cope with the demands of the day. It concentrates on the neck and head – the areas that suffer most. Plenty of water to drink, and plenty of sleep (if possible) complete the cure.

The massage can be given to someone who is fully clothed, and oil is not strictly necessary. If possible, roll a plastic bag of ice in a towel to slip under the sufferer's neck and place cotton wool pads, cooled in iced water, over the eyes.

Quantity of oil required: 5ml (1tsp) of an oil for the face, *see page 11*

1 Cup hands, one on top of the other, over the forehead and gently press down. Count 10, relax for 5, and repeat. Firmly stroke the forehead upwards. Place hands down the sides of the head and press firmly. Count 10, relax for 5 and repeat. Slide hands, palms up, under nape of neck and gently lift to stretch the neck without lifting the head. Hold for 10.

2 Firmly stroke the forehead up from brows with the fingers, one hand following the other. At each sixth stroke slide fingers out over the eyebrows and press gently in over the temples. Then rhythmically stroke the brow upwards with the palms for several minutes.

3 With your fingers stiffly bent, rake the whole scalp from all round the hairline to crown. Then gently tug sections of hair, holding close to the roots, over whole scalp. Finish with long, slow finger strokes through scalp that end by gently pulling the hair away from the head.

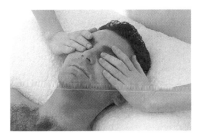

4 Place palms across the forehead, fingertips touching above the nose and slowly slide hands down so that middle and ring fingers are over the eyelids. Press gently for 8, then slide fingers out across eyes to temples. With the first two fingers of each hand gently press and make circles to rotate skin. Finally place tips of index fingers over inner eye corners and hold for 5.

5 Knead tops of each shoulder muscle in turn between the thumbs and fingers of both hands, working out from neck to arm top. Then palm in across shoulder from arm and up to ear with both hands in a flowing movement.

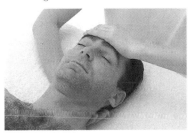

6 Place right hand, palm up, across under neck and gently knead and press in along base of skull. Place left hand across brow and press down gently as you lift neck with right hand (*above*). Hold for 5. Relax. Finish with soothing palm strokes up forehead, getting slower and slower.

Massage to Soothe a Baby

Babies really respond to touch, and this massage is pleasurable for parent and baby alike. After the baby is four weeks old, she can be massaged at any time – not just when she needs soothing, but also as a different way of giving a loving touch. If she is tired the stroking may well send her straight to sleep, and if she is fretful it should help to calm her. Talk to her as you massage and hold her close so that she feels snug and secure.

Keep the baby warm throughout, and find a comfortable position for yourself. Have tissues or towelling to hand in case of accidents. It goes without saying that all strokes should be extra-light, with no downward pressure.

Quantity of oil required: 5ml (1tsp) of an oil for the face, *see page 11*

1 Begin by bending over the baby, resting your arms along the sides of her body. Place your palms over her ears with the fingertips meeting on top of her head. Look at her, talk to her, then gently stroke the forehead back to the crown.

2 Rub a little oil into your hands and place one hand across the top of her forehead, thumb one side fingers the other. Stroke her head to the crown. Then place your palms each side of the face and stroke them up to the top of the head.

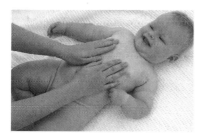

3 Add a little more oil and place your hands over the baby's shoulders. Stroke down over chest, tummy, thighs, legs and feet in light, flowing movements (*above*). Cover the lower body and do a series of shoulder to tummy strokes, one hand following the other rhythmically.

4 With one hand following the other, make the lightest possible circles sweeping in a clockwise direction round the navel from the abdomen. Then sit comfortably and pick up the baby, cradling her side-on against your heart.

5 With your free arm stroke down the baby's side from head to foot, starting with your hand on the head, and using your wrist and arm as part of the stroke. Repeat the step on the baby's other side, holding her the other way around.

6 Lean back comfortably and rest the baby, front down, along your chest. Add more oil if needed and stroke from the shoulders, down the back, over the bottom and down to the toes in continuous sweeps.

7 Cover the baby to keep her warm. Cuddle her to your chest with one hand and use the other to cradle her head and gently stroke it from the top down to the nape of the neck. Finish by sitting up slightly and bending up your knees to support the baby's back as you wrap her up. Support her head at the back with one hand and her back with the other and enjoy a quiet time together.

Massage for a Child's Tummy Ache

To cure a child's tummy ache with this massage, use only the lightest, slowest strokes, keep the movements simple, use plenty of oil, and do lots of repetitions. And put a warm, wrapped, hot water bottle on the area afterwards to keep the muscles relaxed. The best way to do the massage is for the child to be lying in bed with you sitting or standing by the side.

Quantity of oil required: 5ml (1 tsp) of an oil for the face, *see page 11*

WARNING

Tummy ache is very common in children, and usually not serious, but you should consult your doctor if you are at all worried or if any of the following occur:
• pain is severe and persists • there is severe pain with vomiting in a baby or toddler
• pain is associated with high temperature (37.8° C/100° F or above)

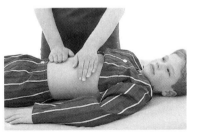

1 Starting with one hand over the solar plexus and the other below the navel, make slow, sweeping circles clockwise round the abdomen. The lower hand moves up and the upper hand down, so that each hand completes a half circle.

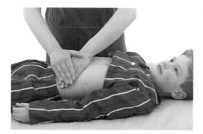

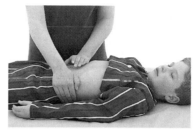

2 Place one hand on top of the other in the middle of the tummy and lightly and rhythmically make clockwise circles round the tummy again. Move out from solar plexus, following base of rib cage, round groin and up and round other side.

3 Place palms side by side over the navel, with fingers covering the solar plexus. Lightly rest for a count of 6, then slide hands apart, out, down and round the lower abdomen.

4 Stroke the sides by placing your hands over one hip, with your fingers tucked under the bottom. Pull one hand after the other firmly but lightly, pulling up towards the tummy. Pull up, do not press in. Repeat on the other side.

5 Cross-stroke over the tummy. Start with right hand over hip as in Step 4 and left hand resting on tummy. Pull up with the right hand and glide across the tummy with your left hand. As hands cross, the left hand should push gently down while the right hand glides over the tummy.

6 Finish with slow cat stroking – a light, flowing stroke with palms down and minimal pressure. Each hand follows the other from the base of the ribs, down the tummy, to the groin. As the lower hand reaches the end of the stroke, curve the palm, so that only the fingertips touch the skin. Make sure the strokes become increasingly slower and lighter.

INDEX

A

Anti-cellulite massage 52-53
Anti-stretch mark massage 49-51

B

Baby, massage for 60-61
Back ache see 28 (lower back ache), 30 (upper back ache)
Beauty massage 46-48
Body massage
  'energizing' 42-43
  'fit for life' 40-41
Body oils 10
Buttocks see 52-53 (anti-cellulite massage)

C

Cellulite, massage to treat 52-53
Child, see 60 (massage for baby), 62 (massage for tummyache)
Circling (massage stroke) 15
Circulation, massage for general 44-45
  legs 35-37
  and see 52 (anti-cellulite massage)

E

Energizing massage 42-43 and see 58 (massage for jetlag)
Equipment for massage 12

F

Face, beauty massage for 46-48
Face oils 11
Feet, massage for 38-39,44-45
Friction rub (massage stroke) 16

H

Hands, massage for 32-34 , 44-45
Hangover, massage for 58-59
Headache
  tension headache 26
  with hangover 58

I

Indigestion see 62 (massage for tummyache)
Insomnia, massage to treat 56-57

J

Jetlag, massage to treat 58-59

K

Kneading (massage stroke) 17
Knuckling (massage stroke) 20

L

Legs, massage for 35-37 and see 52 (anti-cellulite massage)
Ling, Per Henrik 6
Lower back ache, massage for 28-29 and see 54 (massage to soothe period pains)

M

Massage
  benefits and uses of 7, 8
  do-s and don't-s 8-9
  history of 6-7
  oils for 10-11
  preparing for 12-13
  strokes 14-23
  tips for giving 9, 12-13

N

Neck, beauty massage for 46-48, and see 24 (massage for a stiff neck 24

O

Oils for massage 10-11

P

Period pains, massage for 54-55
Pregnancy, massage for 49-51 and see 28 (lower backache)
Pressing (massage stroke) 23
Pummelling (massage stroke) 19

R

Raking (massage stroke) 18

S

Safety advice 8-9
Sleep, massage to induce 56
Stiff neck, massage for 24
Stretch marks, preventing 49
Stretching (massage stroke) 22
Strokes for massage 13, 14-23
Stroking (massage stroke) 14
Swedish massage 6

T

Techniques of massage 13
  and see Circling, Friction rub, Kneading, Knuckling, Pressing, Pummelling, Raking, Stretching, Stroking, Thumbing
Tension
  in hands 32
  in neck 24
  in upper back 30
Tension headache, massage for 26-27
Thumbing (massage stroke) 21
Tummy ache, massage for 62-63

U

Upper back ache, massage for 30-31

W

Wrists, massage for 32-34